25 Resistance Band Workouts:

Low-impact, short, effective workouts for small spaces (including travel!)

TABLE OF CONTENTS

Routine 1: Low-Impact Full Body
Routine 2: Full Body Burn
Routine 3: Core and Lower Body Blast
Routine 4: Upper Body Sculpt
Routine 5: Total Body Tone
Routine 6: Core Stability Circuit
Routine 7: Endurance Booster
Routine 8: Dynamic Strength Builder
Routine 9: Lower Body Burn
Routine 10: Upper Body Pump
Routine 11: Core and Stability Challenge
Routine 12: Full Body Sculpt
Routine 13: Total Body Blast
Routine 14: Full Body Toning
Routine 15: Cardio Blast with Resistance Band
Routine 16: Full Body Burnout
Routine 17: Strength and Stability Circuit
Routine 18: Core and Cardio Fusion
Routine 19: Lower Body Burn
Routine 20: Upper Body Sculpt
Routine 21: Full Body Power
Routine 22: Core and Stability Challenge
Routine 23: Core Stability and Strength
Routine 24: Total Body Blast
Routine 25: Functional Strength and Mobility
BONUS: Cardio and Core Burn

THE BENEFITS

Resistance band training offers numerous health and fitness benefits, making it a versatile and effective form of exercise for individuals of all fitness levels.

Portable and Convenient: Resistance bands are lightweight, compact, and easy to transport, making them ideal for home workouts, travel, or exercising on the go. They can be easily stored in a small bag or suitcase, allowing you to maintain your fitness routine from any location.

Versatility: With resistance bands, you can target every major muscle group in your body, including arms, chest, back, shoulders, legs, and core. From bicep curls to squats to lateral raises, there's a wide range of exercises you can perform with resistance bands to achieve a full-body workout.

Adjustable Resistance: Resistance bands come in various levels of resistance, from light to heavy, allowing you to customize your workout intensity based on your fitness level and goals. You can easily increase or decrease the resistance by adjusting the length of the band or using multiple bands simultaneously.

Joint-Friendly: Unlike some forms of weightlifting that put stress on joints and tendons, resistance band training provides a smooth and controlled resistance throughout the entire range of motion. This makes it a safer option for individuals with joint pain or mobility issues, as well as those recovering from injuries.

Improved Strength and Muscle Tone: Regular resistance band workouts can help increase muscle strength and definition. By challenging your muscles with resistance, you stimulate muscle growth and development, leading to improved muscle tone and overall strength.

Enhanced Functional Strength: Resistance band exercises often mimic natural movement patterns, such as pushing, pulling, and lifting. This helps improve functional strength, which translates to better performance in everyday activities, such as lifting groceries, climbing stairs, or playing sports.

Stability and Balance: Many resistance band exercises require you to engage your core muscles for stability and balance. This helps strengthen the muscles that support your spine and improve overall balance, reducing the risk of falls and injuries, especially as you age.

Affordability: Compared to expensive gym memberships or bulky fitness equipment, resistance bands are an affordable option for anyone looking to add strength training to their fitness routine. A quality set of resistance bands is relatively inexpensive and can last for years with proper care.

Suitable for All Fitness Levels: Whether you're a beginner or an experienced athlete, resistance bands can be tailored to your fitness level and goals. Beginners can start with lighter resistance bands and gradually progress to heavier ones as they build strength and endurance.

Incorporates Variety and Creativity: With resistance bands, you're not limited to traditional weightlifting exercises. There are endless variations and combinations you can explore to keep your workouts interesting and challenging. From compound movements to isolation exercises, you can continuously mix things up to prevent boredom and plateauing.

THE BAND

The resistance band described for these workouts should be a long, elastic band typically made of latex or similar materials. It usually comes in various resistance levels, ranging from light to heavy, allowing users to adjust the intensity of their exercises.

Some bands have handles at each end to provide a secure grip during exercises, but these are not necessary. The handles may have padding or be made of durable materials for comfort and longevity. Some resistance bands also come with ankle straps or door anchors, which can expand the variety of exercises you can perform. Alternatively, you can use a simple resistance band from a physical therapist without any handles or straps. This would be the easiest to pack for travel.

For the workout routines described, a medium resistance band is suitable for most people, but you can adjust the resistance level based on your fitness level and strength. The band should be long enough to allow for full range of motion during exercises like squats and rows, and sturdy enough to provide ample resistance without snapping or breaking.

When selecting a resistance band, ensure it's in good condition with no signs of wear or tear. It's important to use the band safely and according to the manufacturer's instructions to avoid injury. As the bands age (or if they're left in the sun or cold) they can get weaker and snap more easily.

The routines below target all major muscle groups and provide a full-body workout using only a resistance band. Adjust the resistance of the band as needed to challenge yourself appropriately.

Enjoy your workouts!

Warm-Up Routine For All Workouts: 5 Minutes

1. **March in Place (1 minute)**
   - Start by standing tall with your feet hip-width apart.
   - Begin marching in place, lifting your knees towards your chest.
   - Swing your arms naturally as you march to engage your upper body.
   - Focus on landing softly and gradually increasing your pace.
2. **Arm Circles (1 minute)**
   - Extend your arms out to the sides at shoulder height.
   - Make small circles with your arms in a forward motion for 30 seconds.
   - Then, reverse the motion and make small circles in a backward motion for another 30 seconds.
   - Keep your shoulders relaxed and focus on increasing the range of motion with each circle.
3. **Hip Circles (1 minute)**
   - Stand with your feet hip-width apart and place your hands on your hips.
   - Begin by rotating your hips in a circular motion, moving clockwise.
   - Perform smooth, controlled circles, focusing on loosening up your hip joints.
   - After 30 seconds, switch to rotating your hips counterclockwise for another 30 seconds.
4. **Leg Swings (1 minute)**
   - Find a sturdy support, such as a wall or chair, to hold onto for balance.
   - Swing one leg forward and backward in a controlled manner, focusing on increasing the range of motion with each swing.
   - Perform 15-20 swings with each leg.
   - Switch sides and repeat the leg swings on the other leg.
5. **Torso Twists (1 minute)**
   - Stand with your feet hip-width apart and extend your arms out to the sides at shoulder height.
   - Twist your torso to one side, bringing your opposite hand towards your back.
   - Return to the center and twist to the other side, reaching with the opposite hand.
   - Continue alternating sides in a rhythmic motion, focusing on loosening up your spine and engaging your core.

This warm-up routine helps to increase blood flow to your muscles, improve joint mobility, and prepare your body for the upcoming workout. Adjust the duration or intensity of each movement based on your fitness level. Enjoy your workout!

Cool-Down Routine For All Workouts: 5 Minutes

1. **Deep Breathing (1 minute)**
   - Find a comfortable standing or seated position.
   - Close your eyes and take slow, deep breaths in through your nose, filling your lungs completely.
   - Exhale slowly through your mouth, releasing any tension or stress with each breath.
   - Focus on relaxing your body and calming your mind with each breath cycle.

2. **Neck Stretch (1 minute)**
   - Sit or stand tall with your shoulders relaxed.
   - Slowly tilt your head to one side, bringing your ear towards your shoulder.
   - Hold the stretch for 15-30 seconds, feeling a gentle stretch along the side of your neck.
   - Repeat on the other side.
   - You can also add a gentle chin tuck by bringing your chin towards your chest to stretch the back of your neck.

3. **Shoulder Stretch (1 minute)**
   - Reach one arm across your body and use your other hand to gently press the arm towards your chest.
   - Hold the stretch for 15-30 seconds, feeling a stretch in your shoulder and upper back.
   - Repeat on the other side.
   - Focus on keeping your shoulders relaxed and your breathing steady throughout the stretch.

4. **Hamstring Stretch (1 minute)**
   - Sit on the ground with one leg extended straight in front of you and the other leg bent.
   - Reach towards your toes with both hands, keeping your back straight.
   - Hold the stretch for 15-30 seconds, feeling a gentle stretch in the back of your thigh.
   - Switch legs and repeat the stretch on the other side.
   - You can also perform this stretch while standing if sitting on the ground is uncomfortable.

5. **Cobra Stretch (1 minute)**
   - Lie face down on the ground with your palms placed near your chest.
   - Press through your hands to lift your chest off the ground, keeping your hips and thighs on the floor.
   - Hold the stretch for 15-30 seconds, feeling a stretch in your chest, shoulders, and abdominals.
   - Slowly lower back down to the ground and relax.

This cool-down routine helps to lower your heart rate, reduce muscle tension, and improve flexibility after your workout. Hold each stretch for 15-30 seconds and remember to breathe deeply and relax into each stretch. Enjoy the relaxation!

The Workouts

Routine 1: Low-Impact Full Body

1. **Squats with Resistance Band**
    - Stand on the resistance band with feet shoulder-width apart.
    - Hold the handles of the band at shoulder height.
    - Squat down, keeping your chest up and back straight, until your thighs are parallel to the ground.
    - Push through your heels to return to the starting position.
    - Repeat for 12-15 reps.
2. **Bent Over Rows**
    - Stand on the resistance band with feet hip-width apart.
    - Hold the handles of the band with an overhand grip.
    - Bend your knees slightly and hinge at the hips, keeping your back straight.
    - Pull the handles towards your lower ribs, squeezing your shoulder blades together.
    - Slowly lower the handles back to the starting position.
    - Repeat for 12-15 reps.
3. **Standing Chest Press**
    - Anchor the resistance band behind you at shoulder height (use a door anchor if available).
    - Hold the handles with an overhand grip and step forward to create tension in the band.
    - Extend your arms forward at chest height, palms facing down.
    - Push the handles forward until your arms are fully extended, then slowly return to the starting position.
    - Repeat for 12-15 reps.
4. **Lateral Raises**
    - Stand on the resistance band with feet hip-width apart.
    - Hold the handles with palms facing inwards, arms by your sides.
    - Lift the handles out to the sides until your arms are parallel to the ground.
    - Keep a slight bend in your elbows and control the movement.
    - Slowly lower the handles back to the starting position.
    - Repeat for 12-15 reps.
5. **Standing Bicep Curls**
    - Stand on the resistance band with feet shoulder-width apart.
    - Hold the handles with an underhand grip, palms facing up.
    - Keep your elbows close to your sides and curl the handles towards your shoulders.
    - Squeeze your biceps at the top of the movement, then slowly lower the handles back to the starting position.
    - Repeat for 12-15 reps.

Routine 2: Full Body Burn

1. **Resistance Band Deadlifts**
   - Stand on the resistance band with feet hip-width apart.
   - Hold the handles with an overhand grip.
   - Hinge at the hips, keeping your back straight, and lower the handles towards the ground.
   - Squeeze your glutes and hamstrings to return to the starting position.
   - Repeat for 12-15 reps.
2. **Overhead Triceps Extension**
   - Stand on the resistance band with feet hip-width apart.
   - Hold one handle with both hands overhead.
   - Keeping your elbows close to your ears, extend your arms upward until they're fully straight.
   - Slowly lower the handles back behind your head, keeping your elbows stationary.
   - Repeat for 12-15 reps.
3. **Standing Oblique Twists**
   - Stand on the resistance band with feet shoulder-width apart.
   - Hold the handles at chest height with both hands.
   - Engage your core and twist your torso to one side, keeping your hips facing forward.
   - Return to the center and twist to the opposite side.
   - Repeat for 12-15 reps on each side.
4. **Standing Shoulder Press**
   - Anchor the resistance band under one foot and hold the handles at shoulder height.
   - Push the handles overhead until your arms are fully extended.
   - Slowly lower the handles back to shoulder height.
   - Repeat for 12-15 reps.
5. **Reverse Lunges with Bicep Curl**
   - Stand on the resistance band with feet hip-width apart.
   - Hold the handles with palms facing up.
   - Step one foot back into a lunge while simultaneously curling the handles towards your shoulders.
   - Push through the front heel to return to the starting position.
   - Repeat on the other leg for 12-15 reps.

Routine 3: Core and Lower Body Blast

1. **Glute Bridges with Resistance Band**
    - Lie on your back with knees bent and feet flat on the floor.
    - Place the resistance band just above your knees.
    - Engage your glutes and lift your hips towards the ceiling.
    - Squeeze at the top, then lower back down with control.
    - Repeat for 12-15 reps.
2. **Standing Side Leg Raises**
    - Stand on one end of the resistance band and hold onto the other end for balance.
    - Lift one leg out to the side, keeping it straight.
    - Lower it back down with control.
    - Repeat for 12-15 reps on each leg.
3. **Plank with Leg Lifts**
    - Start in a plank position with the resistance band looped around your ankles.
    - Lift one leg off the ground, keeping it straight and in line with your body.
    - Lower it back down and repeat with the other leg.
    - Continue alternating for 12-15 reps on each leg.
4. **Standing Abduction**
    - Stand on one end of the resistance band and hold onto the other end for balance.
    - Lift one leg out to the side against the resistance of the band.
    - Slowly return to the starting position.
    - Repeat for 12-15 reps on each leg.
5. **Russian Twists with Resistance Band**
    - Sit on the floor with knees bent and feet lifted off the ground.
    - Hold the resistance band with both hands in front of your chest.
    - Twist your torso to one side, bringing the band with you.
    - Return to the center and twist to the other side.
    - Repeat for 12-15 reps on each side.

Routine 4: Upper Body Sculpt

1. **Push-ups with Resistance Band**
   - Loop the resistance band around your back and hold one end in each hand.
   - Get into a push-up position with hands slightly wider than shoulder-width apart.
   - Lower your chest towards the ground while keeping tension on the band.
   - Push back up to the starting position.
   - Repeat for 10-12 reps.
2. **Seated Rows**
   - Sit on the floor with legs extended and loop the resistance band around your feet.
   - Hold one end of the band in each hand with arms extended in front of you.
   - Pull the bands towards your torso, squeezing your shoulder blades together.
   - Slowly release back to the starting position.
   - Repeat for 12-15 reps.
3. **Tricep Kickbacks**
   - Stand on the resistance band with feet hip-width apart.
   - Hold the handles with palms facing up, elbows bent at 90 degrees.
   - Straighten your arms behind you, keeping your elbows stationary.
   - Slowly bend your elbows to return to the starting position.
   - Repeat for 12-15 reps.
4. **Bent-over Reverse Flyes**
   - Stand on the resistance band with feet hip-width apart.
   - Hinge at the hips, keeping your back flat, and hold the handles in front of you.
   - Lift the handles out to the sides, squeezing your shoulder blades together.
   - Slowly lower the handles back to the starting position.
   - Repeat for 12-15 reps.
5. **Bicep Curls with Resistance Band**
   - Stand on the resistance band with feet shoulder-width apart.
   - Hold the handles with palms facing up and arms extended down.
   - Curl the handles towards your shoulders, keeping elbows close to your sides.
   - Slowly lower the handles back to the starting position.
   - Repeat for 12-15 reps.

Routine 5: Total Body Tone

1. **Lateral Band Walks**
    - Place the resistance band around your ankles.
    - Take small steps to the side, maintaining tension on the band.
    - Perform 10 steps to the right, then 10 steps to the left.
2. **Resistance Band Squat to Overhead Press**
    - Stand on the resistance band with feet shoulder-width apart.
    - Hold the handles at shoulder height.
    - Perform a squat, then press the handles overhead as you return to standing.
    - Repeat for 12-15 reps.
3. **Single-Leg Romanian Deadlift**
    - Stand on the resistance band with feet hip-width apart.
    - Hold the handles in each hand.
    - Shift your weight onto one leg and hinge forward at the hips, extending the other leg behind you.
    - Keep your back flat and return to standing.
    - Repeat for 10-12 reps on each leg.
4. **Resistance Band Push-up with Row**
    - Loop the resistance band around your back and hold one end in each hand.
    - Get into a push-up position with hands slightly wider than shoulder-width apart.
    - Perform a push-up, then immediately pull one handle towards your ribcage in a row motion.
    - Alternate rows between each push-up.
    - Repeat for 10-12 reps on each side.
5. **Standing Woodchoppers**
    - Anchor the resistance band at shoulder height (use a door anchor if available).
    - Stand sideways to the anchor point with feet shoulder-width apart.
    - Hold the handle with both hands at one side of your body.
    - Rotate your torso and pull the handle diagonally across your body, ending overhead.
    - Slowly return to the starting position.
    - Repeat for 12-15 reps on each side.

Routine 6: Core Stability Circuit

1. **Plank with Shoulder Taps**
   - Get into a plank position with the resistance band looped around your wrists.
   - Keep your body in a straight line from head to heels.
   - Tap one shoulder with the opposite hand while maintaining stability.
   - Return to the starting position and alternate sides.
   - Perform 10 taps on each shoulder.
2. **Dead Bug**
   - Lie on your back with knees bent and feet lifted off the floor.
   - Hold the resistance band with both hands, arms extended towards the ceiling.
   - Extend your right arm overhead and your left leg out straight.
   - Return to the starting position and switch sides.
   - Perform 12-15 reps on each side.
3. **Seated Russian Twists**
   - Sit on the floor with knees bent and feet lifted off the ground.
   - Hold the resistance band with both hands in front of your chest.
   - Lean back slightly and twist your torso to one side, then the other.
   - Keep your core engaged throughout the movement.
   - Perform 12-15 twists on each side.
4. **Mountain Climbers with Resistance Band**
   - Get into a plank position with the resistance band looped around your ankles.
   - Drive one knee towards your chest, then quickly switch legs.
   - Continue alternating legs at a quick pace while maintaining good form.
   - Perform 20 mountain climbers (10 on each leg).
5. **Side Plank with Leg Lift**
   - Get into a side plank position with the resistance band looped around your ankles.
   - Lift your top leg towards the ceiling while keeping your core engaged and hips lifted.
   - Lower your leg back down with control.
   - Perform 10 leg lifts on each side.

Routine 7: Endurance Booster

1. **Resistance Band Squat Jumps**
   - Stand on the resistance band with feet shoulder-width apart.
   - Hold the handles at shoulder height.
   - Perform a squat, then explode upwards into a jump.
   - Land softly and immediately go into the next squat.
   - Repeat for 10-12 reps.
2. **Resistance Band Push-up with Rotation**
   - Loop the resistance band around your back and hold one end in each hand.
   - Get into a push-up position with hands slightly wider than shoulder-width apart.
   - Lower your chest towards the ground, then push back up.
   - At the top of the push-up, rotate your torso and reach one arm towards the ceiling.
   - Return to the push-up position and repeat on the other side.
   - Perform 10-12 reps, alternating sides.
3. **Resistance Band Bent-over Rows**
   - Stand on the resistance band with feet hip-width apart.
   - Hold the handles with palms facing towards each other.
   - Hinge at the hips, keeping your back flat, and bend your knees slightly.
   - Pull the handles towards your lower ribs, squeezing your shoulder blades together.
   - Slowly lower the handles back to the starting position.
   - Repeat for 12-15 reps.
4. **Resistance Band Bicycle Crunches**
   - Lie on your back with knees bent and feet lifted off the ground.
   - Hold the resistance band with both hands, arms extended overhead.
   - Bring one knee towards your chest while simultaneously twisting your torso to bring the opposite elbow towards the knee.
   - Switch sides in a pedaling motion, keeping your core engaged.
   - Perform 20-30 bicycle crunches.
5. **Resistance Band Lateral Raises**
   - Stand on the resistance band with feet hip-width apart.
   - Hold the handles with palms facing inwards, arms by your sides.
   - Lift the handles out to the sides until your arms are parallel to the ground.
   - Keep a slight bend in your elbows and control the movement.
   - Slowly lower the handles back to the starting position.
   - Repeat for 12-15 reps.

Routine 8: Dynamic Strength Builder

1. **Resistance Band Squats with Shoulder Press**
   - Stand on the resistance band with feet shoulder-width apart.
   - Hold the handles at shoulder height.
   - Perform a squat, then press the handles overhead as you return to standing.
   - Lower the handles back to shoulder height and repeat.
   - Do 12-15 reps.
2. **Resistance Band Romanian Deadlifts**
   - Stand on the resistance band with feet hip-width apart.
   - Hold the handles with palms facing towards your body.
   - Hinge at the hips, keeping your back straight, and lower the handles towards the ground.
   - Squeeze your glutes and hamstrings to return to the starting position.
   - Repeat for 12-15 reps.
3. **Resistance Band Chest Flyes**
   - Anchor the resistance band behind you at chest height (use a door anchor if available).
   - Hold the handles with palms facing each other.
   - Step forward to create tension in the band and extend your arms out to the sides.
   - Bring your arms together in front of your chest, squeezing your chest muscles.
   - Slowly return to the starting position.
   - Do 12-15 reps.
4. **Resistance Band Russian Twists**
   - Sit on the floor with knees bent and feet lifted off the ground.
   - Hold the resistance band with both hands in front of your chest.
   - Lean back slightly and twist your torso to one side, then the other.
   - Keep your core engaged throughout the movement.
   - Do 12-15 twists on each side.
5. **Resistance Band Pull-Aparts**
   - Stand on the resistance band with feet shoulder-width apart.
   - Hold the band with both hands in front of you at chest height.
   - Pull the band apart, bringing your hands out to the sides.
   - Squeeze your shoulder blades together at the end of the movement.
   - Slowly return to the starting position.
   - Do 12-15 reps.

Routine 9: Lower Body Burn

1. **Resistance Band Sumo Squats**
   - Stand on the resistance band with feet wider than shoulder-width apart and toes pointed out.
   - Hold the handles with palms facing each other at chest height.
   - Squat down, keeping your chest up and back straight, until your thighs are parallel to the ground.
   - Push through your heels to return to the starting position.
   - Do 12-15 reps.
2. **Resistance Band Deadlifts**
   - Stand on the resistance band with feet hip-width apart.
   - Hold the handles with palms facing towards your body.
   - Hinge at the hips, keeping your back straight, and lower the handles towards the ground.
   - Squeeze your glutes and hamstrings to return to the starting position.
   - Do 12-15 reps.
3. **Resistance Band Side Leg Raises**
   - Attach one end of the resistance band to a sturdy anchor at ankle height.
   - Stand sideways to the anchor point and loop the other end around your ankle.
   - Lift your leg out to the side against the resistance of the band.
   - Slowly return to the starting position.
   - Do 12-15 reps on each side.
4. **Resistance Band Glute Kickbacks**
   - Attach one end of the resistance band to a sturdy anchor at ankle height.
   - Loop the other end around your ankle and face away from the anchor point.
   - Kick your leg back behind you, engaging your glutes.
   - Slowly return to the starting position.
   - Do 12-15 reps on each side.
5. **Resistance Band Calf Raises**
   - Stand on the resistance band with feet hip-width apart.
   - Hold the handles with palms facing towards your body.
   - Lift your heels off the ground, rising onto the balls of your feet.
   - Lower your heels back down.
   - Do 15-20 reps.

Routine 10: Upper Body Pump

1. **Resistance Band Chest Press**
   - Anchor the resistance band behind you at chest height (use a door anchor if available).
   - Hold the handles with palms facing forward at shoulder height.
   - Step forward to create tension in the band and extend your arms forward until they are fully extended.
   - Bring your hands back together, squeezing your chest muscles.
   - Slowly return to the starting position.
   - Do 12-15 reps.
2. **Resistance Band Lat Pulldowns**
   - Anchor the resistance band overhead (use a door anchor if available).
   - Hold the handles with palms facing forward and arms extended overhead.
   - Pull the handles down towards your chest, squeezing your shoulder blades together.
   - Slowly return to the starting position.
   - Do 12-15 reps.
3. **Resistance Band Shoulder Press**
   - Stand on the resistance band with feet hip-width apart.
   - Hold the handles with palms facing forward at shoulder height.
   - Press the handles overhead until your arms are fully extended.
   - Slowly lower the handles back to shoulder height.
   - Do 12-15 reps.
4. **Resistance Band Bicep Curls**
   - Stand on the resistance band with feet hip-width apart.
   - Hold the handles with palms facing up and arms extended down.
   - Curl the handles towards your shoulders, keeping elbows close to your sides.
   - Slowly lower the handles back to the starting position.
   - Do 12-15 reps.
5. **Resistance Band Tricep Extensions**
   - Stand on the resistance band with feet hip-width apart.
   - Hold one handle with both hands overhead.
   - Keeping your elbows close to your ears, extend your arms upward until they are fully straight.
   - Slowly lower the handles back behind your head.
   - Do 12-15 reps.

Routine 11: Core and Stability Challenge

1. **Resistance Band Plank Walks**
     - Get into a plank position with the resistance band looped around your wrists.
     - Walk your hands out to one side, then back to the center, and repeat on the other side.
     - Keep your core engaged and hips stable throughout.
     - Perform 10 steps to each side.
2. **Resistance Band Mountain Climbers**
     - Get into a plank position with the resistance band looped around your ankles.
     - Drive one knee towards your chest, then quickly switch legs.
     - Continue alternating legs at a quick pace while maintaining good form.
     - Perform 20 mountain climbers (10 on each leg).
3. **Resistance Band Bicycle Crunches**
     - Lie on your back with knees bent and feet lifted off the ground.
     - Hold the resistance band with both hands, arms extended overhead.
     - Bring one knee towards your chest while simultaneously twisting your torso to bring the opposite elbow towards the knee.
     - Switch sides in a pedaling motion, keeping your core engaged.
     - Perform 20-30 bicycle crunches.
4. **Resistance Band Russian Twists**
     - Sit on the floor with knees bent and feet lifted off the ground.
     - Hold the resistance band with both hands in front of your chest.
     - Lean back slightly and twist your torso to one side, then the other.
     - Keep your core engaged throughout the movement.
     - Perform 12-15 twists on each side.
5. **Resistance Band Plank Leg Lifts**
     - Get into a plank position with the resistance band looped around your ankles.
     - Lift one leg off the ground, keeping it straight and in line with your body.
     - Lower it back down and repeat with the other leg.
     - Continue alternating legs while maintaining stability.
     - Perform 12-15 leg lifts on each leg.

Routine 12: Full Body Sculpt

1. **Resistance Band Squats with Overhead Press**
   - Stand on the resistance band with feet shoulder-width apart.
   - Hold the handles at shoulder height.
   - Perform a squat, then press the handles overhead as you return to standing.
   - Lower the handles back to shoulder height and repeat.
   - Do 12-15 reps.
2. **Resistance Band Bent-over Rows**
   - Stand on the resistance band with feet hip-width apart.
   - Hold the handles with palms facing towards your body.
   - Hinge at the hips, keeping your back flat, and bend your knees slightly.
   - Pull the handles towards your lower ribs, squeezing your shoulder blades together.
   - Slowly lower the handles back to the starting position.
   - Do 12-15 reps.
3. **Resistance Band Reverse Lunges**
   - Stand on the resistance band with feet hip-width apart.
   - Hold the handles with palms facing towards your body.
   - Step one foot back into a lunge, bending both knees to 90-degree angles.
   - Push through the front heel to return to the starting position.
   - Repeat on the other leg.
   - Do 12-15 reps on each leg.
4. **Resistance Band Chest Flyes**
   - Anchor the resistance band behind you at chest height (use a door anchor if available).
   - Hold the handles with palms facing each other.
   - Step forward to create tension in the band and extend your arms out to the sides.
   - Bring your arms together in front of your chest, squeezing your chest muscles.
   - Slowly return to the starting position.
   - Do 12-15 reps.
5. **Resistance Band Russian Twists**
   - Sit on the floor with knees bent and feet lifted off the ground.
   - Hold the resistance band with both hands in front of your chest.
   - Lean back slightly and twist your torso to one side, then the other.
   - Keep your core engaged throughout the movement.
   - Do 12-15 twists on each side.

Routine 13: Total Body Blast

1. **Resistance Band Squats with Front Raise**
   - Stand on the resistance band with feet shoulder-width apart.
   - Hold the handles with palms facing down and arms extended down in front of you.
   - Perform a squat, then as you return to standing, lift your arms straight out in front of you to shoulder height.
   - Lower your arms back down as you squat again.
   - Repeat for 12-15 reps.

2. **Resistance Band Bent-Over Rows with Twist**
   - Stand on the resistance band with feet hip-width apart.
   - Hold the handles with palms facing each other and arms extended down in front of you.
   - Hinge forward at the hips, keeping your back flat.
   - Pull the handles towards your ribcage, squeezing your shoulder blades together.
   - As you pull, rotate your torso to one side, then return to the center as you lower the handles.
   - Alternate sides with each row.
   - Repeat for 12-15 reps.

3. **Resistance Band Reverse Lunges with Woodchop**
   - Stand on the resistance band with feet hip-width apart.
   - Hold one handle with both hands at your right hip.
   - Step your left foot back into a reverse lunge as you bring the handle diagonally across your body, ending overhead to the left.
   - Return to standing as you lower the handle back to your right hip.
   - Repeat on the other side, alternating sides with each lunge.
   - Repeat for 12-15 reps on each side.

4. **Resistance Band Chest Press with Leg Lower**
   - Lie on your back with knees bent and feet flat on the floor.
   - Hold the handles with palms facing each other and arms extended towards the ceiling.
   - Lower one leg towards the ground as you press the handles up towards the ceiling.
   - Return to starting position as you bring the leg back up.
   - Repeat with the other leg.
   - Alternate legs with each chest press.
   - Repeat for 12-15 reps on each leg.

5. **Resistance Band Plank Rows**
   - Get into a plank position with the resistance band looped around your wrists.
   - Pull one handle towards your ribcage, keeping your elbow close to your body.
   - Lower the handle back to the ground and repeat with the other arm.
   - Continue alternating arms for 12-15 reps on each side.

Routine 14: Full Body Toning

1. **Resistance Band Squat to Overhead Press**
   - Stand on the resistance band with feet shoulder-width apart.
   - Hold the handles at shoulder height.
   - Perform a squat, then press the handles overhead as you return to standing.
   - Lower the handles back to shoulder height and repeat.
   - Do 12-15 reps.

2. **Resistance Band Bent-Over Rows**
   - Stand on the resistance band with feet hip-width apart.
   - Hold the handles with palms facing towards your body.
   - Hinge at the hips, keeping your back flat, and bend your knees slightly.
   - Pull the handles towards your lower ribs, squeezing your shoulder blades together.
   - Slowly lower the handles back to the starting position.
   - Do 12-15 reps.

3. **Resistance Band Reverse Lunges**
   - Stand on the resistance band with feet hip-width apart.
   - Hold the handles at shoulder height.
   - Step one foot back into a lunge while simultaneously lowering the handles towards the ground.
   - Push through the front heel to return to the starting position.
   - Repeat on the other leg.
   - Do 12-15 reps on each leg.

4. **Resistance Band Chest Flyes**
   - Anchor the resistance band behind you at chest height (use a door anchor if available).
   - Hold the handles with palms facing each other.
   - Step forward to create tension in the band and extend your arms out to the sides.
   - Bring your arms together in front of your chest, squeezing your chest muscles.
   - Slowly return to the starting position.
   - Do 12-15 reps.

5. **Resistance Band Russian Twists**
   - Sit on the floor with knees bent and feet lifted off the ground.
   - Hold the resistance band with both hands in front of your chest.
   - Lean back slightly and twist your torso to one side, then the other.
   - Keep your core engaged throughout the movement.
   - Do 12-15 twists on each side.

Routine 15: Cardio Blast with Resistance Band

1. **Resistance Band Jumping Jacks**
    - Stand on the resistance band with feet together and hold the handles in each hand by your sides.
    - Jump your feet out to the sides while raising your arms overhead.
    - Quickly jump your feet back together while lowering your arms.
    - Continue jumping jacks for 1 minute.
2. **Resistance Band High Knees**
    - Stand on the resistance band with feet hip-width apart.
    - Hold the handles at waist height.
    - Drive one knee up towards your chest while pulling the corresponding handle down towards your hip.
    - Quickly switch legs, alternating knees and handles at a fast pace.
    - Continue high knees for 1 minute.
3. **Resistance Band Butt Kicks**
    - Stand on the resistance band with feet hip-width apart.
    - Hold the handles at waist height.
    - Kick your heels up towards your glutes while pulling the corresponding handle towards your hip.
    - Alternate legs at a quick pace, keeping your arms and legs moving.
    - Continue butt kicks for 1 minute.
4. **Resistance Band Skaters**
    - Stand on the resistance band with feet hip-width apart.
    - Hold the handles at waist height.
    - Jump to one side, landing on one foot while crossing the other leg behind you.
    - Swing the opposite arm across your body.
    - Quickly jump to the other side, alternating sides at a fast pace.
    - Continue skaters for 1 minute.
5. **Resistance Band Burpees**
    - Stand on the resistance band with feet hip-width apart.
    - Hold the handles at shoulder height.
    - Squat down, place your hands on the floor, and jump your feet back into a plank position.
    - Perform a push-up, then jump your feet back towards your hands.
    - Explosively jump up, reaching the handles overhead.
    - Repeat burpees for 1 minute.

Routine 16: Full Body Burnout

1. **Resistance Band Squat to Shoulder Press**
   - Stand on the resistance band with feet shoulder-width apart.
   - Hold the handles at shoulder height.
   - Perform a squat, then press the handles overhead as you return to standing.
   - Lower the handles back to shoulder height and repeat.
   - Do 12-15 reps.
2. **Resistance Band Bent-Over Rows**
   - Stand on the resistance band with feet hip-width apart.
   - Hold the handles with palms facing towards your body.
   - Hinge at the hips, keeping your back flat, and bend your knees slightly.
   - Pull the handles towards your lower ribs, squeezing your shoulder blades together.
   - Slowly lower the handles back to the starting position.
   - Do 12-15 reps.
3. **Resistance Band Reverse Lunges with Bicep Curl**
   - Stand on the resistance band with feet hip-width apart.
   - Hold the handles with palms facing up.
   - Step one foot back into a lunge while simultaneously curling the handles towards your shoulders.
   - Push through the front heel to return to the starting position.
   - Repeat on the other leg.
   - Do 12-15 reps on each leg.
4. **Resistance Band Chest Press**
   - Anchor the resistance band behind you at chest height (use a door anchor if available).
   - Hold the handles with palms facing forward at shoulder height.
   - Step forward to create tension in the band and extend your arms forward until they are fully extended.
   - Bring your hands back together, squeezing your chest muscles.
   - Slowly return to the starting position.
   - Do 12-15 reps.
5. **Resistance Band Russian Twists**
   - Sit on the floor with knees bent and feet lifted off the ground.
   - Hold the resistance band with both hands in front of your chest.
   - Lean back slightly and twist your torso to one side, then the other.
   - Keep your core engaged throughout the movement.
   - Do 12-15 twists on each side.

Routine 17: Strength and Stability Circuit

1. **Resistance Band Front Squats**
   - Stand on the resistance band with feet shoulder-width apart.
   - Hold the handles at shoulder height with palms facing in.
   - Perform a squat, keeping your chest up and back straight, until your thighs are parallel to the ground.
   - Push through your heels to return to the starting position.
   - Do 12-15 reps.
2. **Resistance Band Single-Leg Deadlifts**
   - Stand on the resistance band with feet hip-width apart.
   - Hold the handles with palms facing your body.
   - Shift your weight onto one leg and hinge forward at the hips, extending the other leg behind you.
   - Keep your back flat and return to standing.
   - Do 10-12 reps on each leg.
3. **Resistance Band Renegade Rows**
   - Get into a plank position with the resistance band looped around your wrists.
   - Keep your body in a straight line from head to heels.
   - Pull one handle towards your ribcage, keeping your elbow close to your body.
   - Lower the handle back down and repeat on the other side.
   - Do 10-12 reps on each side.
4. **Resistance Band Standing Twists**
   - Stand on the resistance band with feet shoulder-width apart.
   - Hold the handles with both hands at chest height.
   - Twist your torso to one side, then back to the center, and repeat on the other side.
   - Keep your core engaged throughout.
   - Do 12-15 twists on each side.
5. **Resistance Band Glute Bridges with Chest Press**
   - Lie on your back with knees bent and feet flat on the floor.
   - Hold the handles with palms facing each other at chest height.
   - Lift your hips towards the ceiling while pressing the handles overhead.
   - Lower your hips and return the handles to chest height.
   - Do 12-15 reps.

Routine 18: Core and Cardio Fusion

1. **Resistance Band Woodchoppers**
   - Stand on the resistance band with feet shoulder-width apart.
   - Hold one handle with both hands at hip height on one side of your body.
   - Rotate your torso and pull the handle diagonally across your body, ending overhead.
   - Control the movement back to the starting position.
   - Do 12-15 reps on each side.
2. **Resistance Band Mountain Climbers**
   - Get into a plank position with the resistance band looped around your ankles.
   - Drive one knee towards your chest, then quickly switch legs.
   - Continue alternating legs at a quick pace while maintaining good form.
   - Perform 20 mountain climbers (10 on each leg).
3. **Resistance Band Russian Twists**
   - Sit on the floor with knees bent and feet lifted off the ground.
   - Hold the resistance band with both hands in front of your chest.
   - Lean back slightly and twist your torso to one side, then the other.
   - Keep your core engaged throughout the movement.
   - Do 12-15 twists on each side.
4. **Resistance Band Bicycle Crunches**
   - Lie on your back with knees bent and feet lifted off the ground.
   - Hold the resistance band with both hands, arms extended overhead.
   - Bring one knee towards your chest while simultaneously twisting your torso to bring the opposite elbow towards the knee.
   - Switch sides in a pedaling motion, keeping your core engaged.
   - Perform 20-30 bicycle crunches.
5. **Resistance Band Burpees**
   - Stand on the resistance band with feet hip-width apart.
   - Hold the handles at shoulder height.
   - Squat down, place your hands on the floor, and jump your feet back into a plank position.
   - Perform a push-up, then jump your feet back towards your hands.
   - Explosively jump up, reaching the handles overhead.
   - Repeat burpees for 1 minute.

Routine 19: Lower Body Burn

1. **Resistance Band Squats**
    - Stand on the resistance band with feet shoulder-width apart.
    - Hold the handles at shoulder height.
    - Perform squats, keeping your chest up and back straight, until your thighs are parallel to the ground.
    - Push through your heels to return to the starting position.
    - Do 12-15 reps.
2. **Resistance Band Deadlifts**
    - Stand on the resistance band with feet hip-width apart.
    - Hold the handles with palms facing your body.
    - Hinge at the hips, keeping your back straight, and lower the handles towards the ground.
    - Squeeze your glutes and hamstrings to return to the starting position.
    - Do 12-15 reps.
3. **Resistance Band Lunges**
    - Stand on the resistance band with feet hip-width apart.
    - Hold the handles with palms facing up.
    - Step one foot back into a lunge, lowering your back knee towards the ground.
    - Push through the front heel to return to the starting position.
    - Repeat on the other leg.
    - Do 12-15 reps on each leg.
4. **Resistance Band Side Leg Raises**
    - Attach one end of the resistance band to a sturdy anchor at ankle height.
    - Stand sideways to the anchor point and loop the other end around your ankle.
    - Lift your leg out to the side against the resistance of the band.
    - Slowly return to the starting position.
    - Do 12-15 reps on each side.
5. **Resistance Band Glute Bridges**
    - Lie on your back with knees bent and feet flat on the floor.
    - Place the resistance band just above your knees.
    - Engage your glutes and lift your hips towards the ceiling.
    - Squeeze at the top, then lower back down with control.
    - Do 12-15 reps.

Routine 20: Upper Body Sculpt

1. **Resistance Band Bent-Over Rows**
    - Stand on the resistance band with feet hip-width apart.
    - Hold the handles with palms facing towards your body.
    - Hinge at the hips, keeping your back flat, and bend your knees slightly.
    - Pull the handles towards your lower ribs, squeezing your shoulder blades together.
    - Slowly lower the handles back to the starting position.
    - Do 12-15 reps.
2. **Resistance Band Chest Press**
    - Anchor the resistance band behind you at chest height (use a door anchor if available).
    - Hold the handles with palms facing forward at shoulder height.
    - Step forward to create tension in the band and extend your arms forward until they are fully extended.
    - Bring your hands back together, squeezing your chest muscles.
    - Slowly return to the starting position.
    - Do 12-15 reps.
3. **Resistance Band Overhead Shoulder Press**
    - Stand on the resistance band with feet hip-width apart.
    - Hold the handles at shoulder height with palms facing forward.
    - Press the handles overhead until your arms are fully extended.
    - Slowly lower the handles back to shoulder height.
    - Do 12-15 reps.
4. **Resistance Band Bicep Curls**
    - Stand on the resistance band with feet hip-width apart.
    - Hold the handles with palms facing up and arms extended down.
    - Curl the handles towards your shoulders, keeping elbows close to your sides.
    - Slowly lower the handles back to the starting position.
    - Do 12-15 reps.
5. **Resistance Band Tricep Extensions**
    - Stand on the resistance band with feet hip-width apart.
    - Hold one handle with both hands overhead.
    - Keeping your elbows close to your ears, extend your arms upward until they are fully straight.
    - Slowly lower the handles back behind your head.
    - Do 12-15 reps.

Routine 21: Full Body Power

1. **Resistance Band Squat Jumps**
   - Stand on the resistance band with feet shoulder-width apart.
   - Hold the handles at shoulder height.
   - Perform a squat, then explode upwards into a jump.
   - Land softly and immediately go into the next squat.
   - Repeat for 12-15 reps.
2. **Resistance Band Push-ups with Rotation**
   - Get into a push-up position with the resistance band looped around your back.
   - Perform a push-up, then rotate your torso and reach one arm towards the ceiling.
   - Return to the starting position and repeat on the other side.
   - Do 10-12 reps, alternating sides.
3. **Resistance Band Standing Rows**
   - Stand on the resistance band with feet hip-width apart.
   - Hold the handles with palms facing towards each other.
   - Pull the handles towards your lower ribs, squeezing your shoulder blades together.
   - Slowly lower the handles back to the starting position.
   - Do 12-15 reps.
4. **Resistance Band Alternating Lunges with Overhead Press**
   - Stand on the resistance band with feet hip-width apart.
   - Hold the handles at shoulder height.
   - Step one foot back into a lunge while pressing the handles overhead.
   - Return to the starting position and repeat on the other side.
   - Do 10-12 reps on each leg.
5. **Resistance Band Russian Twists**
   - Sit on the floor with knees bent and feet lifted off the ground.
   - Hold the resistance band with both hands in front of your chest.
   - Lean back slightly and twist your torso to one side, then the other.
   - Keep your core engaged throughout the movement.
   - Do 12-15 twists on each side.

Routine 22: Core and Stability Challenge

1. **Resistance Band Plank with Leg Lifts**
   - Get into a plank position with the resistance band looped around your ankles.
   - Engage your core and lift one leg off the ground, keeping it straight.
   - Hold for a moment, then lower it back down.
   - Repeat with the opposite leg.
   - Do 12-15 leg lifts on each leg.
2. **Resistance Band Russian Twists**
   - Sit on the floor with knees bent and feet lifted off the ground.
   - Hold the resistance band with both hands in front of your chest.
   - Lean back slightly and twist your torso to one side, then the other.
   - Keep your core engaged throughout the movement.
   - Do 15-20 twists on each side.
3. **Resistance Band Bicycle Crunches**
   - Lie on your back with knees bent and feet lifted off the ground.
   - Hold the resistance band with both hands, arms extended overhead.
   - Bring one knee towards your chest while simultaneously twisting your torso to bring the opposite elbow towards the knee.
   - Switch sides in a pedaling motion, keeping your core engaged.
   - Do 20-30 bicycle crunches.
4. **Resistance Band Plank with Shoulder Taps**
   - Get into a plank position with the resistance band looped around your wrists.
   - Keep your body in a straight line from head to heels.
   - Tap one shoulder with the opposite hand while maintaining stability.
   - Return to the starting position and alternate sides.
   - Do 12-15 taps on each shoulder.
5. **Resistance Band Mountain Climbers**
   - Get into a plank position with the resistance band looped around your ankles.
   - Drive one knee towards your chest, then quickly switch legs.
   - Continue alternating legs at a quick pace while maintaining good form.
   - Do 20-30 mountain climbers.

Routine 23: Core Stability and Strength

1. **Resistance Band Plank with Shoulder Taps**
   - Get into a plank position with the resistance band looped around your wrists.
   - Keep your body in a straight line from head to heels.
   - Tap one shoulder with the opposite hand while maintaining stability.
   - Return to the starting position and alternate sides.
   - Perform 10 taps on each shoulder.
2. **Resistance Band Bicycle Crunches**
   - Lie on your back with knees bent and feet lifted off the ground.
   - Hold the resistance band with both hands, arms extended overhead.
   - Bring one knee towards your chest while simultaneously twisting your torso to bring the opposite elbow towards the knee.
   - Switch sides in a pedaling motion, keeping your core engaged.
   - Perform 20-30 bicycle crunches.
3. **Resistance Band Russian Twists**
   - Sit on the floor with knees bent and feet lifted off the ground.
   - Hold the resistance band with both hands in front of your chest.
   - Lean back slightly and twist your torso to one side, then the other.
   - Keep your core engaged throughout the movement.
   - Perform 12-15 twists on each side.
4. **Resistance Band Leg Raises**
   - Lie on your back with legs straight and the resistance band looped around your feet.
   - Keep your lower back pressed into the floor as you lift your legs towards the ceiling.
   - Slowly lower them back down without letting them touch the ground.
   - Perform 12-15 leg raises.
5. **Resistance Band Plank Hip Dips**
   - Get into a plank position with the resistance band looped around your wrists.
   - Engage your core and glutes, then slowly lower one hip towards the ground.
   - Return to the starting position and repeat on the other side.
   - Alternate sides for 12-15 reps on each side.

Routine 24: Total Body Blast

1. **Resistance Band Squat to Overhead Press**
   - Stand on the resistance band with feet shoulder-width apart.
   - Hold the handles at shoulder height.
   - Perform a squat, then press the handles overhead as you return to standing.
   - Lower the handles back to shoulder height and repeat.
   - Do 12-15 reps.
2. **Resistance Band Deadlifts**
   - Stand on the resistance band with feet hip-width apart.
   - Hold the handles with palms facing towards your body.
   - Hinge at the hips, keeping your back straight, and lower the handles towards the ground.
   - Squeeze your glutes and hamstrings to return to the starting position.
   - Do 12-15 reps.
3. **Resistance Band Bent-Over Rows**
   - Stand on the resistance band with feet hip-width apart.
   - Hold the handles with palms facing towards your body.
   - Hinge at the hips, keeping your back flat, and bend your knees slightly.
   - Pull the handles towards your lower ribs, squeezing your shoulder blades together.
   - Slowly lower the handles back to the starting position.
   - Do 12-15 reps.
4. **Resistance Band Push-ups**
   - Get into a push-up position with the resistance band looped around your back.
   - Perform push-ups, keeping your body in a straight line from head to heels.
   - Engage your core and chest muscles as you lower and raise your body.
   - Do 10-12 reps.
5. **Resistance Band Plank with Leg Lifts**
   - Get into a plank position with the resistance band looped around your ankles.
   - Lift one leg off the ground, keeping it straight and in line with your body.
   - Hold for a moment, then lower it back down and lift the other leg.
   - Continue alternating legs for 12-15 reps on each leg.

Routine 25: Functional Strength and Mobility

1. **Resistance Band Squat to Overhead Reach**
    - Stand on the resistance band with feet hip-width apart.
    - Hold the handles with palms facing each other at shoulder height.
    - Perform a squat, then as you return to standing, press the handles overhead.
    - Reach as high as you can while keeping the arms straight.
    - Return to the starting position and repeat for 12-15 reps.
2. **Resistance Band Bent-Over Reverse Flyes**
    - Stand on the resistance band with feet hip-width apart.
    - Hold the handles with palms facing each other, arms extended towards the floor.
    - Hinge at the hips, keeping the back flat, and slightly bend the knees.
    - Raise your arms out to the sides, squeezing your shoulder blades together.
    - Slowly lower the handles back to the starting position.
    - Do 12-15 reps.
3. **Resistance Band Romanian Deadlifts**
    - Stand on the resistance band with feet hip-width apart.
    - Hold the handles with palms facing your body.
    - Hinge at the hips, keeping the back straight, and lower the handles towards the ground.
    - Squeeze your glutes and hamstrings to return to the starting position.
    - Do 12-15 reps.
4. **Resistance Band Standing Rotations**
    - Stand on the resistance band with feet shoulder-width apart.
    - Hold the handles together in front of your chest with both hands.
    - Rotate your torso to one side, keeping your hips facing forward.
    - Return to the center and repeat on the other side.
    - Do 12-15 reps on each side.
5. **Resistance Band Glute Bridges with Hip Abduction**
    - Lie on your back with knees bent and feet flat on the floor.
    - Place the resistance band just above your knees.
    - Lift your hips towards the ceiling while pushing your knees outward against the resistance band.
    - Squeeze at the top, then lower back down with control.
    - Do 12-15 reps.

BONUS Routine: Cardio and Core Burn

1. **Resistance Band Jumping Jacks**
   - Stand on the resistance band with feet together and hold the handles in each hand by your sides.
   - Jump your feet out to the sides while raising your arms overhead.
   - Quickly jump your feet back together while lowering your arms.
   - Continue jumping jacks for 1 minute.
2. **Resistance Band Plank Jacks**
   - Get into a plank position with the resistance band looped around your ankles.
   - Jump both feet out to the sides, then back together.
   - Keep your core engaged and hips stable throughout.
   - Perform plank jacks for 1 minute.
3. **Resistance Band Bicycle Crunches**
   - Lie on your back with knees bent and feet lifted off the ground.
   - Hold the resistance band with both hands, arms extended overhead.
   - Bring one knee towards your chest while simultaneously twisting your torso to bring the opposite elbow towards the knee.
   - Switch sides in a pedaling motion, keeping your core engaged.
   - Perform bicycle crunches for 1 minute.
4. **Resistance Band Mountain Climbers**
   - Get into a plank position with the resistance band looped around your ankles.
   - Drive one knee towards your chest, then quickly switch legs.
   - Continue alternating legs at a quick pace while maintaining good form.
   - Perform mountain climbers for 1 minute.
5. **Resistance Band Russian Twists**
   - Sit on the floor with knees bent and feet lifted off the ground.
   - Hold the resistance band with both hands in front of your chest.
   - Lean back slightly and twist your torso to one side, then the other.
   - Keep your core engaged throughout the movement.
   - Perform Russian twists for 1 minute.

Printed in Dunstable, United Kingdom